Vegan

Your Step-by-Step Guide to a Healthy Fat-Free
Lifestyle

(Simple and Delicious Everyday Recipes)

Martin Bown

Published by Robert Satterfield Publishing House

Vegan Diet: Your Step-by-Step Guide to a Healthy Fat-Free Lifestyle (Simple and Delicious Everyday Recipes)

ISBN 978-1-989682-75-3

Legal & Disclaimer

The information contained in this book is not designed to replace or take the place of any form of medicine or professional medical advice. The information in this book has been provided for educational and entertainment purposes only.

TABLE OF CONTENT

Part 1

Introduction

This book contains proven steps and strategies on how to cook delicious and healthy vegan dishes. If you are put off with the idea of going vegan, this cookbook will be a great help for you. Some people frown at the thought of going full vegan because they are often confronted with false impressions such as vegan dishes are nothing but a bunch of boring green leafy veggies, fruits, and tofu-based chows.

This book will show you a good number of vegan recipes that are easy to make, budget-friendly, and 100% vegan. This includes breakfast recipes, lunch and dinner recipes, smoothies and flavored water, and vegan snacks. With the willingness to try more whole food and lead a healthier lifestyle, you can easily whip great vegan food that are healthy and incredibly delicious.

Thanks again for getting this book. I hope you enjoy it!

CHAPTER 1: The Vegan Diet: An Overview

The vegan diet is considered to be the kindest diet ever existed for two reasons: this diet has zero animal products, meaning there is no animal who suffered for the sake of giving you food on the table. And second, for the rest of your life, you will be consuming plant-based food and enjoy plant nutrients considered vital in your goal to living a healthy and long life.

The vegan diet is strictly plant-based. It prohibits consumption of meat. Apart from that, it also excludes by-products of animals such as eggs, cheese and milk, and other milk-producing animals, butter, and honey from bees.

Many people thought the vegan diet is something that is highly restrictive and hard to follow. But with the right planning and guidance from professionals, this diet can be sustainable and easy to follow.

As the vegan diet becomes restrictive of nutrients such as protein, iron, and vitamin B12 all found in animal products, most vegans get these said nutrients from beans, soy products, and lentils. It is also recommended to take food supplements to keep the body and its different systems function well.

Vegan Diet and Weight Loss

Veganism is a lifestyle choice. Most people turn to this kind of diet to primarily lose weight. However, you must keep in mind of the following:

Read food labels when going grocery shopping

Veganism takes dedication, lots of patience, and practice. Successful vegans are able to maintain their lifestyle because they choose to make their own meals so they will have full control of the kind of ingredients they add and adhere to the right cooking methods. Therefore, when going grocery shopping, make sure to opt for organic produce. Read the labels carefully as some vegan-safe products may contain animal-based ingredients.

Veganism is not about consuming more soy-based products

Soy-based products are made especially for vegans, but if you have adrenal or thyroid gland problems, increasing your soy intake is not recommended. People with bleeding disorders and/or those who have recently undergone major surgery are advised to do away with soy as this could lead to delay healing and blood clotting. With these said, it is all the more important to consult your health care provider before you embark on the vegan diet.

Not all vegan food are healthy

One of the biggest misconceptions about veganism is that they are all healthy and good for the body. Although you are going plant-based, remember that the method of cooking should be considered. Take for example deep frying vegan vegetables such as sweet potatoes, kale, and spinach. Cooking them this way could lead to bad cholesterol and ultimately weight gain because of the creation of fat cells or adipose tissues. So if you have finally committed yourself to going vegan, make sure that you keep a careful eye at the cooking methods or do the cooking yourself. When dining out, opt for vegan dishes that are lightly cooked, steamed, boiled, and grilled.

Here is a list of food to avoid and those that you can store in your pantry:

Food to avoid

- Red meat such as lamb and sheep, beef, goat, cold cuts, pork cuts, and other exotic animals.
- White meat such as chicken, duck, quail meat and eggs, turkey, seafood, fish, and shellfish.

Food to store in your pantry

- Fresh produce such as fresh fruits, vegetables, herbs, and beans.

- Canned/bottled beans, fruits, and vegetables.

- Dried pulses and grains such as lentils, nuts, and dried beans.

- Non-dairy alternatives such as nut butter, nut cheeses, or soy-based margarine, almond milk, quinoa milk, and oat milk among others.

- Mushrooms

- Organic Herbs and spices

In the succeeding chapters, you will get to know different vegan recipes that are easy to do. Most of the recipes can be "made ahead" so you could store them, refrigerate or freeze, and then quickly reheat and serve.

CHAPTER 2: Vegan Breakfast Recipes

1. Vegan Cardamom Pancakes

Ingredients:

- 1 cup all-purpose flour
- 2 tablespoons coconut oil
- ½ teaspoon baking powder
- ½ teaspoon baking soda
- ¼ tsp. cardamom powder
- 2 tablespoons muscovado sugar
- 1 teaspoon apple cider vinegar
- 1 cup coconut milk
- ¼ cup chocolate buttons
- ¼ tsp. vanilla extract

Directions:

In a large bowl, combine all-purpose flour, coconut oil, baking powder, baking soda, cardamom powder, muscovado sugar, apple cider vinegar, coconut milk, chocolate buttons, and vanilla extract. Stir but do not over mix.

Lightly grease a skillet and set over medium heat. Divide the batter into equal portions. Pour into the hot skillet.

When edges are set, flip to the other side. Do not press down on pancakes. Sprinkle brown sugar on top. Serve.

2. Breakfast Fried Rice

Ingredients:

- 1 tablespoon olive oil
- 2 garlic cloves, minced
- 2 leeks
- 3 cups cooked brown rice
- 1 tablespoon onion powder
- 1 cup frozen mixed vegetables (corn, peas, and carrots), thawed
- Pinch of salt
- Pinch of pepper

Directions:

In a pan, heat the oil. Sauté garlic and onions for 3 minutes until translucent and fragrant. Add in the leeks. Cook for another 3 minutes.

Add the cooked rice, onion powder, mixed vegetables, salt, and pepper. Stir-fry until all the ingredients are mixed well and the rice is heated through.

Adjust seasoning. Divide into equal portions. Serve.

3. Strawberry Chocolatey Pancakes

Ingredients:
- 2 tablespoons coconut oil, melted
- 1 tablespoon baking powder
- 1 cup whole wheat flour, finely milled
- 1 cup coconut milk
- 2 tablespoons palm sugar, crumbled
- ½ cup chocolate buttons, vegan-safe
- 1 teaspoon vanilla extract
- Pinch of salt
- 4 pieces fresh strawberries, diced

Directions:

In a mixing bowl, combine the baking powder, whole wheat flour, coconut milk, palm sugar, chocolate buttons, vanilla extract, and salt. Stir but do not over mix. Fold in the strawberries.

Meanwhile, grease the pan over medium heat. Divide batter into equal portions. Pour into the hot pan.

When edges are set, flip to the other side. Do not press down on pancakes. Sprinkle brown sugar on top. Serve.

4. Broccoli and Cauliflower Mix

Ingredients:
- 1 tablespoon olive oil
- 2 garlic cloves, minced
- 1 onion, minced
- 1 red bell pepper, deseeded and cubed
- 2 heads broccoli, sliced into small florets
- 2 heads cauliflower, sliced into small florets
- 2 tablespoons vegetable stock

- Pinch of salt
- Pinch of pepper

Directions:

In a pan, heat the oil. Sauté garlic and onions for 3 minutes until translucent and fragrant.

Add the red bell pepper, broccoli and cauliflower florets, vegetable stock, salt, and pepper. Cook until the broccoli turns a shade brighter.

Adjust seasoning. Divide into equal portions. Serve.

5. Mix Veggie Fritters

Ingredients:
- 1 teaspoon garlic powder
- 1 onion, peeled, minced
- ½ cup carrot, processed
- 1 cup squash, processed
- ½ cup sweet potato, processed
- Pinch of salt
- Pinch of pepper

- olive oil

Directions:

In a bowl, combine the garlic powder, carrot, squash, sweet potato, salt, and pepper. Mix well. Roll mixture into balls; slightly flatten balls.
Pour olive oil into a pan over medium heat. Fry veggie fritters until crisp and golden brown. Drain on paper towels. Serve.

6. Breakfast Pumpkin Fritters
Ingredients:

- 1 can pumpkin puree
- 1 carrot, grated
- ¼ cup almond flour
- ¼ cup fresh chives, minced
- ¼ teaspoon red pepper flakes
- Dash cumin powder
- Dash nutmeg powder
- Pinch of salt
- Pinch of pepper
- olive oil

Directions:

In a bowl, combine pumpkin puree, carrots, almond flour, chives, red pepper flakes, cumin nutmeg, salt, and pepper. Mix well. Roll mixture into balls; slightly flatten balls.
Pour olive oil into a pan over medium heat. Fry pumpkin fritters until crisp and golden brown. Drain on paper towels. Serve.

7. Coconut Porridge with Raisins and Apricots

Ingredients:
- ½ cup coconut milk
- 1 ½ cups water
- ¼ cup rolled oats
- 1 large banana, mashed
- 1 teaspoon raisins
- ½ teaspoon dried apricots, chopped
- 1 teaspoon pure maple syrup
- 1 teaspoon desiccated coconut

Directions:

In an ovenproof dish, combine the coconut milk, water, oats, mashed banana, apricots, raisins, and maple syrup. Stir and bring to a boil.

Allow to simmer for 10 minutes. Adjust seasoning, if needed.

Ladle portions of porridge into bowls. Garnish with coconut. Serve.

8. Banana-Walnuts Pancakes

Ingredients:

- 2 tablespoon olive oil
- 1 tablespoon baking powder
- 1 cup whole wheat flour, finely crushed
- 1 cup coconut milk
- 1 overripe bananas, mashed
- ½ cup toasted walnuts, chopped
- 1 teaspoon vanilla extract

- Pinch of salt
- 2 tablespoon pure maple syrup

Directions:

In a large bowl, combine baking powder, whole wheat flour, coconut milk, bananas, walnuts, vanilla extract, and salt. Mix well. Meanwhile, grease the pan with olive oil over medium heat. Divide the batter into equal portions. Pour into the hot pan.
When edges are set, flip to the other side. Do not press down on pancakes. Drizzle with maple syrup. Serve.

9. Pumpkin Pancakes with Chocolates

Ingredients:
- 2 tablespoons coconut oil, melted
- 1 tablespoon baking powder
- 1 cup whole wheat flour, finely crushed
- 1 teaspoon pumpkin pie spice
- 1 teaspoon vanilla extract
- 1 cup coconut milk
- ½ cup canned pumpkin puree

- ½ cup chocolate buttons
- Pinch of salt
- Maple syrup

Directions:

In a large bowl, combine coconut oil, baking powder, wheat flour, palm sugar, pumpkin pie spice, vanilla extract, coconut milk, pumpkin puree, chocolate buttons, and salt.

Meanwhile, grease the pan with oil over medium heat. Divide the batter into equal portions. Pour mixture into the hot pan.

When edges are set, flip to the other side. Do not press down on pancakes. Drizzle with maple syrup. Serve.

10. Peanut Butter Pumpkin Pancakes

Ingredients:

- 1 tablespoon baking powder
- 2 tablespoons coconut oil, melted
- 1 cup coconut milk

- 1 cup whole wheat flour, finely crushed
- ½ cup canned pumpkin puree
- ¼ cup peanut butter buttons
- ¼ cup chocolate buttons
- 1 teaspoon vanilla extract
- Pinch of salt
- 2 tablespoons palm sugar, crumbled

Directions:

In a large bowl, combine baking powder, coconut oil, coconut milk, whole wheat flour, pumpkin puree, peanut butter buttons, chocolate buttons, vanilla extract, and salt. Do not over mix.

Meanwhile, grease the pan with oil over medium heat. Divide the batter into equal portions. Pour mixture into the hot pan.

When edges are set, flip to the other side. Do not press down on pancakes. Drizzle with palm sugar. Serve.

11. Breakfast Coriander Bread

Dry Ingredients:

- 2 teaspoon active dry yeast
- 4 cups whole wheat flour, unbleached and finely crushed
- 1 teaspoon white sugar
- Pinch of salt

Wet Ingredients:

- 2 tablespoons coconut oil
- 2 cups boiled water
- 1 teaspoon vinegar
- 1 teaspoon coriander seeds
- ⅛ cup fresh coriander, minced

Directions:

In a large bowl, combine the dry yeast, wheat flour, white sugar, and salt. Make a well in the center and then pour coconut oil, water, vinegar, coriander seeds.

Mix until the dough comes together. Turn out the dough on a floured surface and make depression in middle. Add the fresh coriander and knead for 10 minutes or until elastic.

Place the dough in the same bowl. Cover the bowl and let it rise in a warm place for 1 hour or until the dough has double in size.

Meanwhile, grease the loaf pans. Punch the dough down and divide the dough in half on a floured surface.

Stretch the dough and tuck in edges underneath. Put in the prepared loaf pans. Let the dough rise for 15 minutes.

Preheat oven to 375°F. Add coriander seeds on top of the dough. Bake for 30 minutes or until golden brown.

Remove from the oven and place on a cooling rack. Remove loaves before slicing.

12. Cornbread

Dry Ingredients:

- 2 cups cornmeal

- 2 cups all-purpose flour
- ½ cup palm sugar, crumbled
- Pinch of salt

Wet Ingredients:

- 2 cups coconut milk
- ½ cup coconut oil, melted
- ½ cup canned whole corn kernels
- 4 flax eggs

Directions:

Preheat the oven to 375°F. Grease the loaf pans with coconut oil.

In a large bowl, combine the cornmeal, all-purpose flour, sugar, and salt. Make a well in the center and then pour the coconut milk, coconut oil, corn kernels, and eggs.

Mix the ingredient until well combined. Pour equal amounts of batter into the loaf pan. Bake for 30 minutes or until an inserted toothpick comes out clean.

Remove from the oven and let cool on the rack. Remove loaves before slicing.

13. Chocolate   Coconut   Porridge   with Cashew Nuts

Ingredients:

- 2 cups water
- ¼ cup rolled oats
- ½ cup coconut milk
- 1 tablespoon cocoa powder
- 1 tablespoon cashew nuts

Directions:

In an oven dish, pour water, rolled oats, coconut milk, and cocoa powder over high heat. Bring to a boil.

Turn down the heat and allow to simmer for 15 minutes. Adjust seasoning.

To serve, ladle equal portions into bowls. Top with cashew nuts. Serve.

14. Blueberry and Lemon Muffins

Dry ingredients

- 2 cups all-purpose flour
- 1 teaspoon baking soda
- 2 teaspoons fresh lemon zest
- Pinch of salt

Wet ingredients
- 1 cup rice milk
- $^1/_3$ cup coconut oil
- 1 tablespoon lemon juice, freshly squeezed
- ¾ cup palm sugar, crumbled

*1 cup fresh blueberries

Directions:

Preheat the oven to 375°F. Line paper liners into the muffin tins.

Meanwhile, in a bowl, put dry and wet ingredients into separate bowls. Pour wet ingredients into dry. Fold in the blueberries.

Spoon equal portions into muffin tins. Bake for 30 minutes or until an inserted toothpick comes out clean.

Remove from the oven and allow the muffins to cool. Serve.

CHAPTER 3: Vegan Lunch and Dinner Recipes

1. Classic Banana, Pineapple, and Mango Salad

Ingredients:

- 1 banana, sliced into thick disks
- 1 can pineapple tidbits, drained
- 1 ripe mango, diced

For the dressing
- ½ cup coconut cream, canned
- 2 tablespoons lime juice, freshly squeezed
- 1 tablespoon white sugar

Directions:

For the dressing, combine coconut cream, lime juice, and white sugar in a bottle with tight lid. Shake the bottle until the sugar dissolves.

In a large salad bowl, combine the banana, pineapple tidbits, and mango. Drizzle the dressing and toss to combine.

Place equal portions into salad bowls. Serve.

2. Mushrooms and Corn Combo

Ingredients:
- 1 tablespoon olive oil
- 1 large onion, minced
- 2 tablespoons vegetable stock
- 1 can button mushrooms
- 2 cans whole corn kernels
- Pinch of salt
- Pinch of pepper

Directions:

Pour olive oil into the pan over medium heat.

Sauté the onion for 3 minutes or until translucent. Add the vegetables stock, button mushrooms, corn kernels, salt, and pepper. Allow to simmer for 15 minutes.

Adjust seasoning. Serve.

3. Green Asparagus Rice

Ingredients:
- 1 tablespoon olive oil
- 2 leeks, sliced diagonally
- 3 cups cooked white rice
- ¼ tablespoon garlic powder
- 1 cup frozen peas, thawed
- 1 handful green asparagus, sliced into ¼ inch long
- ½ piece ripe avocado, diced
- Pinch of salt
- Pinch of pepper
- 2 teaspoons sesame seeds, toasted

Directions:

Pour olive oil into the pan over medium heat.

Sauté leeks for 4 minutes or until tender. Add the cooked rice, garlic powder, peas, asparagus, avocado, salt, and pepper. Continue stirring until the ingredients are

well combined and the rice is heated through.
Adjust seasoning. Divide into equal portions and sprinkle sesame seeds and leeks. Serve.

4. Fully Loaded Beans Casserole

Ingredients:
- 4 cups mushroom stock
- 1 onion minced
- 1 carrot, diced
- 1 red bell pepper, diced
- 1 cup dried black beans
- 1 cup dried pinto beans
- 1 teaspoon oregano powder
- Pinch of salt
- Pinch of pepper
- 1 can peeled tomatoes

Directions:

Pour the stock, onion, carrots, red bell pepper, black beans, pinto beans, oregano powder, salt, and pepper into slow cooker set over medium heat. Secure the lid.

Cook for 4 hours or until the beans are tender. Stir in the tomatoes. Allow 15 more minutes for the tomatoes to blend well with the dish.

Ladle equal portions into bowls. Serve.

5. Grapes, Apples, and Nuts Salad

Ingredients:

- 4 green grapes seedless, halved
- 4 red grapes, seedless, halved
- 2 baby carrots, thinly shaved
- 2 apples, cubed
- ¼ cup cashew nuts
- ¼ teaspoon honey

Directions:

In a salad bowl, combine green and red grapes, carrots, apples, and cashew nuts. Toss well to combine.

Place equal portions into salad bowls. Drizzle with honey. Serve.

6. Spicy White Bean

Ingredients:

- 3 garlic, minced
- 1 piece white onion, minced
- ½ teaspoon liquid smoke hickory seasoning
- 4 cups boiled water
- 2 cups dried white beans
- banana chili, minced
- 1½ tablespoon chili powder
- 1½ tablespoon cumin powder
- Pinch of salt
- 1 can canned tomatoes peeled and diced
- 1 ½ tablespoon tomato paste

Directions:

In a slow cooker over medium heat, put the garlic, onions, smoke hickory seasoning, water, white beans, banana chili, chili powder, cumin powder, and salt. Secure the lid.

Cook for 4 hour or until the beans are tender. Turn off heat and add the tomatoes and tomato paste. Allow 15 more minutes for the tomatoes and paste to blend well with the dish.

Ladle recommended serving into bowls. Serve.

7. Yellow Yam Noodles

Ingredients:

- 1 piece yellow yam, quartered lengthwise
- Pinch of salt
- water

Directions:

Scrape cut the side of the yam using a vegetable peeler until you have a pile of noodles.

Submerge vegetable noodles in the water for 20 minutes and rinse well. Drain.

Place the yam and salt into the colander. Toss well to combine. Allow to drain for 20 minutes. Shake off for excess moisture.
Damp and layer on tea towel to remove more moisture and salt. Remove vegetable noodles from tea towel. Use or store in a container.

8. Vegan Zucchini Noodles

Ingredients:
- 2 large zucchini, deseeded
- Pinch of salt

Directions:

Make deep scores on one side of the zucchini.
Scrape cut the side of the yam using a vegetable peeler until you have a pile of noodles.
Place the yam and salt into the colander. Toss well to combine. Allow to drain for 20 minutes. Shake off for excess moisture.

Damp and layer on tea towel to remove more moisture and salt. Remove vegetable noodles from tea towel. Use or store in a container.

9. Pizza Loaf

Dry Ingredients:
- 4 cups whole wheat flour, finely grated
- 2 ½ teaspoon active dry yeast
- 1 teaspoon white sugar
- 1 teaspoon salt

Wet Ingredients:
- 2 cups boiled water
- 4 tablespoons olive oil, divided

- ¼ cup sun-dried tomatoes, minced
- ⅛ teaspoon dried basil leaves
- ⅛ teaspoon dried rosemary leaves

Directions:

In a mixing bowl, combine wheat flour, active yeast, sugar, and salt. Meanwhile, in a separate bowl, mix the egg and half of the olive oil. Make a well in the center. Pour in the wet ingredients onto the well.

Mix until the dough comes together. Turn out the dough on a floured surface and make depression in middle. Add the sun-dried tomatoes, basil, and rosemary and knead for 10 minutes or until elastic.

Lightly grease (same) bowl with oil. Place dough in. Cover bowl with saran wrap. Let dough rise in a warm place for 1 to 1½ hours, or until double in size.

Lightly grease bread loaf pans. Place the dough in the same bowl. Cover the bowl and let it rise in a warm place for 1 hour or until the dough has double in size.

Meanwhile, grease the loaf pans. Punch the dough down and divide the dough in half on a floured surface.

Preheat the oven to 375°F. Bake for 25 minutes. Remove from the oven and put on the cooling rack. Remove from the oven and place on a cooling rack. Remove loaves before slicing.

Use loaf to make your own homemade vegan pizza.

10. Cauliflower and Rice Porridge

Ingredients:

- ¼ teaspoon olive oil
- 1 garlic clove, minced
- 2 leeks, minced
- 2 cups vegetable stock
- 1 head cauliflower, sliced into florets
- ½ cup uncooked brown rice
- 1 tablespoon cashew nuts, roughly chopped
- 1 teaspoon curry powder
- Pinch of salt
- Pinch of black pepper

Directions:

Pour olive oil into a pan over medium heat.

Sauté garlic and leeks for 3 minutes until tender and fragrant.

Pour the stock, cauliflower, brown rice, cashew nuts, curry powder, salt, and pepper.
Allow to simmer for 15 minutes. Adjust seasoning
Ladle equal portions into bowls.

CHAPTER 4 Vegan Smoothies and Fruity Infusions

1. Pineapple and Pear Smoothie

Ingredients:

- 2 cups fresh pineapples, chopped
- 1 pear, quartered
- 2 cups crushed ice
- 1 tablespoon green *stevia*

Directions:

Put the pineapples, pear, crushed ice, and stevia in a blender. Blend until smooth. Pour into a glass and serve.

2. Raisins and Apples Flavored Water

Ingredients:

- 6 cups water
- 1 cup raisins
- 1 lime, sliced into wedges
- 2 red apples, cored, diced
- 1 dried cinnamon bark, whole

Directions:

Pour water and add raisins, lime, red apples and cinnamon bark in a large pitcher. Chill in the fridge for 3 hours.
Stir using a muddler for the fruits to further release their flavor. Strain infusions directly into glasses. Serve.

3. Strawberry and Black Currants Flavored Water

Ingredients:
- 6 cups water
- 4 pieces fresh strawberries, quartered
- 2 cups fresh black currants
- 1 celery stalk

Directions:

Pour water and add strawberries, black currants, and celery stalk in a large pitcher. Chill in the fridge for 3 hours.

Stir using a muddler for the fruits to further release their flavor. Strain infusions directly into glasses. Serve.

4. Kale and Bananas Smoothie

Ingredients:
- 1 cup coconut milk
- 2 cups kale leaves
- 2 bananas, frozen and chopped
- 2 cups crushed ice
- 1 tablespoon frozen blueberries, thawed

Directions:

In a blender, pour coconut milk and add the kale leaves, bananas, and crushed ice. Blend until smooth.

Pour into glasses. Garnish with blueberries on top. Serve.

5. Berries Overload Flavored Water

Ingredients:

- 4 cups water
- 2 cups fresh coconut water
- ½ cup strawberries, quartered
- 1 cup green grapes, halved
- 1 cup red grapes, halved

Directions:

Pour water and coconut water. Add strawberries, and green and red grapes in a large pitcher. Chill in the fridge for 3 hours.

Stir using a muddler for the fruits to further release their flavor. Strain infusions directly into glasses. Serve.

6. Sweet Grapes and Orange Flavored Water

Ingredients:

- 6 cups water
- 3 cup red sweet grapes, halved
- 1 pear, cored, quartered
- 1 orange, sliced into wedges

Directions:

Pour water and stir in the grapes, pear, and orange in a large pitcher. Chill in the fridge for 3 hours.

Stir using a muddler for the fruits to further release their flavor. Strain infusions directly into glasses. Serve.

CHAPTER 5

Vegan Snacks

1. Homemade Tahini

Ingredients:

- 4 tablespoons extra virgin olive oil
- 1 cup sesame seeds, raw
- Pinch of salt

Directions:

Pour olive oil, sesame seeds, and salt into
the blender. Process until smooth.
Adjust seasoning. Spread on toast.

2. Chickpea Salad Sandwich

Ingredients:
- 1 slice whole wheat bread, toasted

For the chickpea salad
- ½ tsp. Tahini paste
- ¼ cup canned chickpeas, mashed
- ¼ cup ripe avocado, mashed
- ¼ teaspoon parsley, minced
- Pinch of salt
- Pinch of pepper

Directions:

In a mixing bowl, combine tahini paste, chickpeas, avocado, parsley, salt, and pepper.

Spread this on top of the bread slice.

Heat in a toaster until warmed through.

Serve.

3. Cashew Pesto and Mushroom

Ingredients:

- 2 slices wheat bread
- 1 tablespoon cashew pesto sauce
- 1 teaspoon olive oil
- 1 fresh porcini mushroom, thinly sliced
- 1 garlic clove, minced
- 1 tablespoon balsamic vinegar
- palm sugar
- Pinch of salt
- Pinch of pepper
- 1 teaspoon parsley, minced

Direction:

Spread pesto sauce on one side of wheat bread. Set aside.

Meanwhile, in a skillet over medium heat, pour the olive oil.

Saute mushrooms until golden brown. Stir in the garlic, balsamic vinegar, sugar, and salt. Stir.

Allow it to simmer for 5 minutes for the mushrooms to cook through. Remove from heat.

Spoon mixture on top of the bread. Drizzle some fresh parsley. Serve.

4. Cherry Tomatoes Spread

Ingredients:
- 1 thick Pizza loaf, toasted
- 1 tablespoon pesto sauce

Toppings

- ¼ teaspoon apple cider vinegar
- ¼ teaspoon balsamic vinegar
- 2 cherry tomatoes, quartered
- Pinch of palm sugar, crumbled
- extra virgin olive

- pinch of salt
- pinch of pepper

Directions:

Spread the pesto sauce on one side the pizza loaf. Heat in the bread toaster until warmed through.

Meanwhile, in a bowl, combine apple cider vinegar, balsamic vinegar, cherry tomatoes, palm sugar, olive oil, salt, and pepper. Toss well to combine.

Spread the mixture on warmed bread. Serve.

4. Roasted Tahini

Ingredients:
- 1 cup sesame seeds
- 4 tablespoons extra virgin olive oil
- Pinch of salt

Directions:

Place the sesame seeds on the skillet over medium heat. Toast until golden and fragrant. Stir continuously to prevent burning seeds.

Let cool completely and then transfer into the blender.

Pour the oil and sprinkle salt. Process until smooth. Spread on toast.

5. Spicy Hummus

Ingredients:

- 2 tablespoons lemon juice, freshly squeezed
- 4 garlic cloves, crushed
- 2 tablespoons roasted tahini
- 1 jalapeno pepper, minced
- 2 tablespoons olive oil
- ¼ teaspoon cumin powder
- 1 can chickpeas
- Pinch of salt
- Pinch of pepper

Directions:

Pour lemon juice and add garlic cloves, roasted tahini, jalapeño pepper, olive oil, cumin powder, chickpeas, salt, and pepper.

Process until smooth. Adjust seasoning. Spread on toast.

6. Spicy Zucchini Bruschetta

Ingredients:
- 1 slice wheat bread
- 1½ tablespoon spicy hummus
- ½ tablespoon pomegranate seeds
- ½ tablespoon tomato, diced
- ½ tablespoon cucumber, diced
- ¼ tablespoon chives, minced
- Pinch of salt
- Pinch of pepper

Directions:

Spread hummus on wheat bread. Heat in the bread toaster until warmed through. Meanwhile, combine pomegranate seeds, tomato, cucumber, chives, salt, and

pepper. Spread this on top of bruschetta.
Serve.

7. Cashew Cheese

Ingredients:
- ¼ cup water
- 2 tablespoons apple cider vinegar
- 2 tablespoons lemon juice, freshly squeezed
- 2 garlic cloves, minced
- 1 tablespoon Dijon mustard
- 1 cup raw cashew nuts
- Pinch of salt
- Pinch of pepper

Directions:
Pour water, apple cider vinegar and lemon juice into the blender. Add the garlic, Dijon mustard, cashew nuts, salt, and pepper Process until smooth.
Spread lightly on toast.

8. Totally Vegan Pizza Slice

Ingredients:

- 1 slice pizza loaf, toasted
- 1 tablespoon tomato pesto sauce
- ½ tablespoon onions, julienned
- ½ tablespoon red bell pepper, julienned
- extra virgin oil
- ½ cup cashew cheese
- Dash of red pepper flakes
- Pinch of pepper

Directions:

Spread tomato pesto sauce on pizza loaf. Layer the onions, and bell pepper.

Drizzle olive oil and put some cashew cheese on top. Season with salt and pepper.

Heat in the bread toaster until warmed through. Serve.

9. Carrots and Cashew Muffins

Ingredients:

- 1½ cups whole wheat flour
- 2 teaspoon baking soda
- 2 flax eggs
- ½ cup white sugar
- ½ cup steel-cut oats
- ¼ cup coconut oil
- 4 carrots, grated
- ¼ cup cashew nuts, chopped
- 1 teaspoon vanilla extract

Directions:

Preheat the oven to 375°F.

Put paper liners in muffin tins.

In a mixing bowl, combine flour, baking soda, eggs, white sugar, oats, coconut oil, grated carrots, cashew nuts, and vanilla extract. Do not over mix.

Spoon equal portions into lined muffin tins. Bake for 25 minutes or an inserted toothpick comes out clean when inserted.

Remove from the oven. Let it cool before removing muffins from tins.

Place the muffins on the cake rack. Serve.

10. Cranberries with Walnuts Muffins

Ingredients:
- 1 ½ cups all-purpose flour
- 2 teaspoon baking powder
- 1⅛ cups walnut milk
- 1 serving flax egg
- ½ cup fresh cranberries
- ¼ cup coconut oil
- ¼ cup walnuts, chopped
- 3 tablespoons palm sugar, crumbled
- ½ teaspoon salt

Directions:

Preheat the oven to 375°F.

Put paper liners in muffin tins.

In a mixing bowl, combine flour, baking powder, walnut milk, flax eggs, cranberries, coconut oil, walnuts, palm sugar, and salt. Do not over mix.

Spoon equal portions into lined muffin tins. Bake for 25 minutes or an inserted toothpick comes out clean when inserted. Remove from the oven. Let it cool before removing muffins from tins.

Place the muffins on the cake rack. Serve.

11. Apples and Grapes Salad

Ingredients:
- 2 apples, diced
- ¼ cup roasted walnuts
- 4 large green grapes, quartered
- 3 teaspoon apple cider vinegar
- 1 teaspoon palm sugar, crumbled
- 1 teaspoon extra virgin olive oil
- Pinch of salt
- Pinch of white pepper

Directions:

In a bottle with tight fitting lid, combine the apples, walnuts, and grapes. Pour apple cider vinegar, sugar, olive oil, salt, and pepper.

Seal and shake the bottle well until sugar and salt dissolves.

Put all the ingredients in a bowl. Drizzle the dressing. Toss well to combine.

Place equal portions into salad bowls. Serve

Conclusion

Thank you again for getting this book!

I hope this book was able to help you gain confidence in eating and making your own vegan meals at home.

Going vegan does not mean you have to eat carrot sticks, cucumber, and leafy greens all the time. In case you did not know, these kinds of food contain as much important vitamins and minerals weigh against store bought eats and fast food chows. These days, it is more practical to cook your own vegan meals that are far healthier, tastier, and are definitely a more economical option.

The next step is to craft your own dishes through the recipes in this eBook and discover vegan meals that you can serve regularly. Who knows, maybe you can even introduce these vegan food to family and friends.

Part 2

Vegan Spicy Chickpeas

Ingredients

1 tablespoon vegetable oil

2 onions, peeled and finely chopped

4 garlic cloves, finely chopped

2 tablespoons minced fresh gingerroot

2 teaspoons ground coriander

1 teaspoon cumin seed

1 teaspoon salt

1/2 teaspoon fresh ground black pepper

1/2 teaspoon cayenne pepper (reduce if that's too spicy for your tastes)

2 teaspoons balsamic vinegar

2 cups coarsely chopped tomatoes (, canned or fresh)

2 (19 ounce) cans chickpeas, rinsed and drained

Directions

In a skillet over medium heat, cook onions, stirring, just until they begin to brown; then add garlic and all spices and cook, stirring, for 1 minute.

Add vinegar and tomatoes and bring to a boil, then place mixture in your slow cooker; add chickpeas and combine well.

Cover and cook on Low for 6 to 8 hours or on High for 3 to 4 hours, or until the mixture is hot and bubbling.

Serve with hot naan or pita bread

Vegan Mango Curry Tofu

Serves:4 servings

Ingredients
TOFU:
14 ounces firm tofu
2 teaspoons safflower or other neutral oil
¼ teaspoon cayenne
¼ teaspoon ground cinnamon
½ teaspoon Garam Masala
¼ teaspoon salt
CURRY:
¾ cup chopped red onion
1 (1-inch) knob of ginger
3 cloves garlic

2 tablespoons water
1 teaspoon safflower or other neutral oil
¼ teaspoon cumin seeds
2 bay leaves
4 cloves
1¼ cups canned or culinary coconut milk
¾ cup ripe mango pulp or puree (unsweetened or lightly sweetened canned)
½ teaspoon salt
2 teaspoons apple cider vinegar
Generous dash of black pepper
¼ teaspoon Garam Masala, for garnish
2 tablespoons chopped cilantro, for garnish

Instructions
Tofu:
Cut the tofu slab into ½-inch slices. Place them on a clean kitchen towel. Cover with another kitchen towel. Place a 10-pound (approximate) weight on top and let sit for 10 minutes. Alternatively, you can use pressed tofu. Cut the tofu slices into ½-inch cubes.

Heat the oil in a large skillet over medium heat. When the oil is hot, tilt the skillet so the oil coats it evenly. Add the tofu and cook until lightly brown on some sides, stirring occasionally, 4 minutes. Add the cayenne, cinnamon, garam masala, and salt and mix well to coat. Cook for another 2 minutes and set aside.

Curry:

In a blender, combine the onion, ginger, and garlic and blend into a smooth puree with 2 tablespoons of water. Heat the oil in a large skillet over medium heat. When the oil is hot, add the cumin seeds, bay leaves, and cloves. Cook for 1 minute.

Add the pureed onion and cook until the onion mixture is dry and does not smell raw. Stir occasionally to avoid sticking, 13 to 15 minutes.Add the coconut milk, mango pulp, salt, and vinegar and mix well. Add the tofu and all the spices from the tofu skillet to the sauce skillet. Add a dash of black pepper.

Mix, cover and cook until the sauce comes to a boil, 5 minutes. Reduce the heat to low and cook uncovered until the sauce thickens and desired consistency is achieved, about 15 minutes. Taste and adjust the salt and tang. Add ½ teaspoon or more sugar if the mango pulp was not sweet. Garnish with cilantro and a dash of garam masala and serve hot.

Vegan Bean & Oat Chili

Ingredients
For The Morning Ingredients:
1 medium sweet potato, unpeeled (if organic)
2 cups (475 ml) water
½ cup (97 g) dry Vaquero or pinto beans
¼ cup (46 g) oat groats (Make sure they are clearly marked gluten-free.)
¼ cup (33 g) diced carrot
¼ cup (38 g) diced bell pepper
2 cloves garlic, minced
½ teaspoon oregano
½ teaspoon chipotle powder
¼ teaspoon turmeric

FOR THE EVENING

INGREDIENTS:

1 cup (56 g) chopped greens

2 tablespoons (32 g) tomato paste

Salt and pepper, to taste

Instructions

Please note this recipe uses a 1½ to 2 quart slow cooker. You can double or triple for a larger slow cooker, but you may need to adjust the liquid up!

In the morning:

Take the sweet potato and poke holes in it with a fork and set aside. Add all the other morning ingredients to your slow cooker. Place the sweet potato on top of the mixture. It will sink into the chili, which is fine. Cook on low for 7 to 9 hours.

About 20 minutes before serving:

Remove the sweet potato and set on a plate. Turn the slow cooker to high. Mix the chili and add a bit more water if it's too dry. Now stir in the greens and tomato paste. Pop the sweet potato back in to keep it hot. Cook for about 20 minutes or until the greens are cooked the way you like them.

Carefully remove the hot sweet potato with tongs, cut it in half, and put each half in its own bowl. Taste the chili and add salt and pepper to suit your taste. Smother each sweet potato half with chili and serve.

RECIPE VARIATIONS

Serve with any of your favorite chili toppings such as vegan sour cream, vegan cheese, hot sauce, etc.

Instead of waiting 20 minutes for the greens and tomato paste to cook, just stir them in and serve. The greens will still cook a bit from the heat of the stew, and if you cut them smaller, the texture will be pretty much the same.

This recipe calls for oat groats, but if you don't have any, feel free to substitute steel-cut oats

Vegan Lentil Soup

Serves 4

Ingredients
1 tablespoon olive oil
1/2 small onion, chopped
2 cloves garlic, minced
1 cup lentils
5 cups water
2 cups potato, chopped
1 carrot, chopped
1 stalk celery, minced
1 tablespoon bouillon
1 sprig fresh rosemary (or 1/4 teaspoon ground)
2 sprigs fresh thyme (or 1 teaspoon dried)
smoked salt (or plain salt) and pepper, to taste

Instructions
The night before: Saute the onion in oil until it turns translucent, then add the garlic and cook one more minute. Store

cooked mixture with other cut veggies in the fridge overnight.

In the morning: Add everything except salt and pepper to the slow cooker. Cook 7 – 9 hours on low.

Before serving: Taste, add salt and pepper. Adjust seasonings if needed.

Veggie Lentil Soup

Ingredients
1 cup dry lentils
1 1/2 cups carrots, chopped
1 1/2 cups celery, chopped
1 1/2 cups onions, chopped
3 garlic cloves, minced
1 teaspoon dried basil
1 teaspoon dried oregano
1/2 teaspoon dried thyme
1 tablespoon dried parsley
2 bay leaves
3 1/2 cups vegetable broth (2 cans)
1 1/2 cups water

1 (14 1/2 ounce) cans diced tomatoes
fresh ground black pepper, to taste

Directions
Rinse lentils.
Place all ingredients except the pepper
into a 4-6 quart slow cooker.
Cover and cook on low for at least 12
hours, or high for at least 5 hours.
Season with pepper and remove the bay
leaves before serving.

Vegan Sweet Potato & Stew Black Bean

Ingredients
2 Tbsp olive oil
2 cups finely chopped onions
2 Tbsp minced fresh ginger root
2 tsp chili powder
1-1/2 tsp ground cumin
1-1/2 pounds red-skinned sweet potatoes
(yams; about 2 medium), peeled, cut into
1/2-inch pieces

1-1/4 cups orange juice

2 Tbsp minced garlic

2 15- to 16-ounce cans black beans, rinsed, drained

1-2 chipotle chiles in adobo, chopped (to taste)

1 red bell pepper, chopped

Kosher salt and fresh black pepper, to taste

Toppings (optional): sour cream, diced avocado, orange or lime wedges

Directions

In a 5- or 6-quart slow cooker, add the olive oil, onions and ginger root. Turn the cooker to HIGH while you prepare the sweet potatoes.

Add the chili powder, cumin, sweet potato pieces, orange juice and garlic. Turn the cooker to LOW, cover, and cook for 3 hours.

After the potatoes have cooked and are nearly tender, stir in the black beans, chipotle chile peppers, bell pepper, and 1/2 teaspoon each of kosher salt and black pepper. Cook on LOW for 1 hour, or until the sweet potatoes are cooked through.

Taste, and adjust seasoning with more salt and pepper, if needed.

Serve hot. Can be made several days ahead.

Black Garbanzo Bean Curry

Ingredients:

1 1/2 cups dried black garbanzo beans (or use regular garbanzo beans, but they will require a few hours longer to cook)

1 small onion, coarsely chopped

1/2 cup chopped fresh tomato (I used cherry tomatoes)

2 tsp. minced ginger root

2 tsp. minced garlic

1/2 - 1 tsp. cayenne pepper (I used 1/2 tsp. and it was very hot so I'm not sure I'd recommend using the full amount unless you really like it spicy!)

1 1/2 tsp. cumin seeds

1/2 tsp. turmeric

1/2 tsp. chile powder

2 tsp. salt (or less)

1 can petite dice tomatoes (optional)

1/2 cup thinly sliced green onions (optional)

3-4 T chopped fresh cilantro

1 T fresh squeezed lemon juice

Instructions:

Pick over the garbanzo beans, removing any broken ones or debris found in the beans, and wash beans if needed.

Using a food processor or the bowl attachment of an immersion blender, puree together the onion, fresh tomatoes, minced ginger, minced garlic, cayenne, cumin seeds, turmeric, chile powder, and salt. Put the paste mixture in the slow cooker with the beans and 4 cups of water and cook on high for about 9 hours, or until beans are soft. (They will still be slightly chewy when they're done. I would start to check after about 6 hours and see if you want to add more water.)

When beans are done, taste for seasoning. You can eat the curry at this point, but it was too spicy for me so I added the can of tomatoes and sliced green onions and cooked for about 1 hour more on high. When it's done to your liking, stir in the chopped cilantro and lemon juice. Serve hot, over brown rice if desired.

Vegan Mexican Bowl

Slow Cooker Ingredients:
1 cup long-grain brown rice
2 cups vegetable stock (I used a can of vegetable broth and a little water to make 2 cups)
1 cup finely chopped onion
1 red bell pepper, chopped small
1 green bell pepper, chopped small
1 can (4 oz.) diced green chiles plus juice (Anaheim chiles, not jalapenos)
2 cans (15 oz.) black beans, rinsed well and drained

salt to taste

Salsa Ingredients:
1/2 cup diced tomato
1 large Poblano pepper, very finely diced
1/2 cup thinly sliced green onion
1/2 cup finely chopped fresh cilantro
1 large avocado (or 2 small avocadoes) cut into cubes about 1 inch
1 T + 2 T fresh lime juice
2 T extra-virgin olive oil
1/2 tsp. ground cumin (or more, to taste)
salt to taste

Instructions:
Combine the rice, vegetable stock, and finely chopped onion in the slow cooker and cook on high for 1 1/2 hours, or until rice is just starting to get tender. While rice cooks, chop the red and green bell pepper, and open the diced green chiles. Drain the black beans into a colander placed in the sink and rinse well with cold water until no more foam appears; then let beans drain well.

After 1 1/2 hours, add the chopped red bell pepper, chopped green bell pepper, diced green chiles with juice, and drained black beans to the slow cooker and gently combine with the rice. Add salt to taste and then cook on high for about 30 minutes more.

While the rice mixture finishes cooking, chop the tomato, cilantro, and Poblano pepper and thinly slice the green onion. Cut the avocado into cubes about 1 inch across and toss in a bowl with 1 T of lime juice. (Use a bowl that will hold all the salsa ingredients. Add the chopped tomato, chopped cilantro, finely chopped Poblano, sliced green onion, other 2 T lime juice, 2 T olive oil, ground cumin, and salt to taste, and gently combine.

The slow cooker mixture is ready when the rice is tender (and preferably the peppers are barely cooked, with still quite a bit of crunch.) Serve hot or warm, with a generous scoop of the Poblano-Avocado

Salsa on top. You could add other toppings such as desired.

Vegetables & Chinese Barbecued Tofu

Ingredients
1 package (about 1 lb.) extra-firm, regular (not silken) tofu
Sauce:
1 small onion, minced
3 cloves garlic, minced
2 teaspoons fresh ginger root, minced
8 ounces no salt added tomato sauce
1/4 cup hoisin sauce
2 tablespoons seasoned rice wine vinegar
1/4 teaspoon vegan Worcestershire sauce
1 tablespoon low sodium soy sauce
1 tablespoon spicy brown mustard
1/4 teaspoon crushed red pepper
2 teaspoons molasses
1/4 teaspoon five spice powder
1/8 teaspoon ground black pepper

salt to taste (optional)
2 tablespoons water
Vegetables:
2-3 stalks broccoli (stalks only; reserve florets for another use)
2 medium zucchini, cut into 1/2-inch cubes
1/2 large red or green bell pepper, cut into 1-inch squares
1 8-ounce can sliced water chestnuts

Instructions

Cut the tofu into 1/2-inch thick slices. Place them on a few paper towels and cover them with 2 or 3 more. Press lightly to remove some of the moisture from the tofu. Cut the slices into triangles or other shapes.

Heat an oiled, non-stick skillet until hot, and place the tofu slices in it. Brown well on both sides. When they are done, place them in a crockpot that has been sprayed with non-stick spray. Set the crockpot to high heat and cover.

Using the same skillet, sauté the onions, garlic, and ginger until the onion softens, about 3 minutes. Add the remaining ingredients and heat, stirring, until bubbly. Pour the sauce over the tofu and stir well to combine. Replace the cover and cook on high for 3 hours.

Prepare the broccoli stalks by trimming off the tough ends and peeling off the outer skin. Slice into 1/4-inch thick rounds. After the tofu has cooked for 3 hours, add the broccoli and other vegetables. Stir well to combine and cover tightly. Cook for about 1 more hour. Vegetables should be tender but not over-cooked. Serve over brown rice. Makes 3-4 servings.

Notes

Cooking options:

If you need to cook the tofu for a longer time, set the cooker on low and add 2 or 3 more tablespoons of water to the sauce. Cook for about 5-6 hours before adding the vegetables. Turn the heat up to high once the veggies are added. Note: This is not a good option for larger crockpots because the volume of food is too low.

To cook this in the oven, preheat to 375 F and put the tofu and sauce into a non-metal baking dish coated with cooking spray. Cook for 30 minutes before adding the vegetables. Cover and cook for about 15 more minutes, until vegetables are just tender.

Try using frozen and defrosted tofu and skip the pan-frying.

Preparation time: 15 minute(s)

Vegan Fiesta Baked Beans

Makes 4-6 servings

Ingredients
1 cup dried pinto beans (or if you want, you can just use a can of beans)
1 (14 oz) can diced tomatoes with juice (or you can use fresh)
1 (4 oz) can green chile peppers
1 tsp minced garlic
1/2 tsp onion powder
Juice of 1 lime, plus more for garnish
1 Tbsp tapioca
Salt and pepper

1/2 cup chopped cilantro
Avocado slices, optional

Instructions

1.Soak your pinto beans in plenty of water overnight. In the morning drain off the water and place beans in a slow cooker. Cover with water about 2 inches above the beans. Cover and cook on HIGH for 3-4 hours or on LOW for 6-8 hours (or until beans are tender). Drain water from beans. Place beans back in slow cooker.

2.Add in the tomatoes, green chiles, garlic, onion powder, lime juice, tapioca, and salt and pepper to taste.

3.Cover and cook on LOW for about 3 hours.

4.Stir in the cilantro and salt and pepper to taste.

5.Serve with avocado and extra lime, if desired.

Vegan Indian Rice Pudding

serves 8

Ingredients

1 cup (185 g) long grain brown rice
6 cups (1448 ml) nondairy milk (I used So Delicious Unsweetened Coconut milk)
1/2 cup (83 g) golden raisins
1/2 cup (73 g) slivered or chopped almonds (pistachios and/or cashews work great too)
1 teaspoon cardamom
sweetener to taste – I used 2 small packets of stevia and about 2 tablespoons of agave nectar – you can use regular sugar, brown rice syrup, etc.

Instructions

Place all the ingredients except for your sweetener of choice into a 3 1/2 to 4 quart slow cooker. (Double the recipe if you have a larger slow cooker.)
Cook on low for 4 to 5 hours or on high for about 2 1/2 hours. The size of your slow cooker and how hot it runs will change the exact cooking time. Add sweetener and

stir in. Then taste and add extra sweetener if you feel that you need it. (If you are using stevia I would recommend adding 1/8 teaspoon at a time. Just a little too much and it becomes bitter.)

The pudding will still be a little loose in the slow cooker. But it will thicken in the fridge. Serve it cold topped with extra raisins and nuts. You could even go crazy and add some fresh berries too!

Lentil Sloppy Joes

Makes 4 cups
Hands-on time: 15 minutes
Time to table: 3 - 8 hours

Ingredients
1 cup (185g/6.5oz) dried brown or green lentils
1-1/2 cups (323g/12oz) vegetable broth
1 15-ounce (425g) can diced tomatoes
1/4 cup + 1 tablespoon (75g/2.5oz) tomato paste

1 onion, chopped fine

1/2 red or green bell pepper, chopped fine

1 tablespoon apple cider vinegar

1 tablespoon minced garlic

1-1/2 teaspoons oregano

1-1/2 teaspoons smoked paprika (don't skip this)

2 teaspoons dried parsley

1 tablespoon chili powder

1 teaspoon kosher salt

Freshly ground black pepper

Cayenne pepper to taste (I used 1/16t)

Instructions

Stir all ingredients together right in the slow cooker. There's no need for measuring cups, just eyeball or get out the kitchen scale for the lentils, broth and tomato paste! Cover and cook on high for 3 - 4 hours or on low for 7 - 8 hours. Check for consistency, it might be necessary to take the lid off for the last 30 minutes or so.

Serve in buns or as a side dish. Keeps for a week or more, easy to rewarm.

Vegan Saag Paneer

Ingredients
4 to 5 large cloves garlic, finely chopped
3 tablespoons ginger root, finely chopped
1½ cups tomato sauce
1 tablespoon garam masala
1 tablespoon ground coriander
1 tablespoon ground cumin
1½ teaspoons salt (separated into 1 tsp and ½ tsp)
⅛ teaspoon cayenne pepper
1 15-ounce can light coconut milk
2 16-ounce bags frozen chopped spinach
1 6-ounce bag baby spinach leaves
2 packages savory marinated tofu (I like the Trader Joe's Organic), cut into cubes
½ cup frozen peas
fresh cilantro, chopped for garnish (optional)

cooked brown rice for serving

Instructions
-Add all ingredients EXCEPT for fresh spinach, tofu, peas and ½ teaspoon of salt to slow cooker
Set to low and cook for 4 hours.
At about 3 hours and 30 minutes, add in fresh spinach and stir
When fresh spinach is wilted, puree entire mixture with a handheld immersion blender until creamy
Next fold in tofu cubes, frozen peas and remaining ½ teaspoon of salt
Put lid back on slow cooker and let tofu and peas warm up.
Serve over brown rice and chopped cilantro.
Keeps well in the fridge for leftovers and freezes great!

Vegan Spicy Pinto Bean

Ingredients

1 Tbsp olive oil
2 medium onions, diced
2 stalks celery, diced
4 cloves garlic, minced
2 tsp ground cumin
1 tsp Mexican oregano
4-oz can chopped green chiles
1 tsp kosher salt
1/2 tsp fresh black pepper
28-oz can chopped or diced tomatoes, with juice (I use POMI)
2 15-oz cans pinto beans, drained and rinsed
2 dried guajillo chile peppers
1 jalapeño pepper, roughly chopped
10-oz bag frozen corn kernels
6 cups chopped kale
Optional toppings (not for vegan version): shredded Cheddar cheese or sour cream
Sliced lime, for garnish

Directions

In a nonstick frying pan, heat the oil over medium heat. Add the onions and celery and cook, stirring a few times, until the onions are soft, 4-5 minutes. Add the garlic, cumin, Mexican oregano, salt, pepper and green chiles, and stir for 1 minute. Add the tomatoes, raise the heat to high, and bring to a boil.

Transfer the tomato mixture to a 5- or 6-quart slow cooker. Add the beans, stir to combine, and cook on LOW for 6 hours.

Meanwhile, 1 hour before the beans finish cooking, heat 2 cups of water in the microwave until it boils, 2-3 minutes on HIGH. Soak the dried guajillo chile peppers for 30 minutes (you might need to put a small plate on top to keep the peppers submerged).

Tear the soaked peppers in pieces (save the soaking liquid), and add them to a small blender along with the jalapeño. Purée, and set aside.

When the beans finish cooking, stir in the chile mixture and the frozen corn. Add the kale in batches, stirring each batch to submerge the leaves as best you can in the tomato sauce. Raise the slow cooker heat to HIGH, and cook for 20-30 minutes, until the kale is tender.

Garnish individual bowls with shredded Cheddar cheese or sour cream (if not vegan), and a squirt of lime. Or, let cool completely, pack into airtight containers, and freeze.

White Bean and Garlic Hummus
Makes about 1 1/2 cups
Ideal slow cooker size: 3 quart

Ingredients
2/3 cup dried white beans, rinsed
6 garlic cloves, peeled
1/4 cup extra virgin olive oil
Juice of 1 lemon
Kosher salt and black pepper, to taste

Directions
1.Place beans in bottom of slow cooker. Add in the garlic cloves.
2.Cover beans with water about 2 inches above the beans.

3.Cover and cook on LOW for about 8 hours or on HIGH for about 4 hours, or until beans are very tender.

4.Pour slow cooker contents into a colander and let all the water drain off. Transfer beans and garlic to a blender.

5.Add in olive oil and lemon juice.

6.Puree until totally smooth.

7.Salt and pepper a little, blend, taste again, salt and pepper again and repeat until you get it perfectly seasoned.

White Bean Soup

Serves: 6-8 (makes 9 cups)

Ingredients
2 Tbsp olive oil $0.32
4 cloves garlic $0.32
1 medium yellow onion $0.73
½ lb. carrots $0.55
4 stalks (1/2 sleeve) celery $0.80
1 lb. dry navy beans* $1.69
1 whole bay leaf $0.15

1 tsp dried rosemary $0.10
½ tsp dried thyme $0.05
½ tsp smoked paprika $0.05
Freshly cracked pepper (15-20 cranks of a mill) $0.05
1½ tsp (or more to taste) salt $0.05

Instructions

Mince the garlic, dice the onion, slice the celery, and slice the carrots into thin rounds. Add the olive oil, garlic, onion, celery, and carrots to a large (5qt or larger) slow cooker.

Sort through the beans and remove any debris or stones. Give them a quick rinse and then add them to the slow cooker, along with the bay leaf, rosemary, thyme, paprika, and some freshly cracked pepper.

Add SIX CUPS of water to the slow cooker and stir to combine the ingredients. Place the lid on the slow cooker and cook for 8 hours on low or on high for 4-5 hours.

After 8 hours, stir the soup and mash the beans slightly. Starting with just a ½ tsp, add salt to your liking. I used about 2 tsp total, but keep tasting and adding more, ½ tsp at a time, until it reaches the level that you prefer.

Vegan White Bean Stew

Serves: 10-12 servings

Ingredients
2 lbs. white beans
2 large carrots, peeled and diced
3 large celery stalks, diced
1 onion, diced
3 cloves garlic, minced or chopped
1 bay leaf
1 tsp. each: dried rosemary, thyme, oregano
10-12 cups water
2 Tbsp. salt (according to taste, can start with 1 Tablespoon and add more at end if needed)
Ground black pepper, to taste
1 large can (28 ounces) diced tomatoes (I like Muir Glen Organic Fire Roasted)

5-6 cups (or more) roughly chopped leafy greens (spinach, chard, kale)
Rice, polenta, or bread for serving

Instructions
Sort through and rinse beans several times in cool water. Add to the slow cooker along with the diced carrots, celery, onions, garlic, bay leaf and dried herbs. Add the water. (Use less for a thicker stew, more for more of a soup.) Cover and cook on high for 3 hours, or low for 6 hours. Remove lid from slow cooker and add the salt and pepper, and diced tomatoes. Let cook for another 1-1½ hours, or until beans are very soft. (If they are already soft after the initial cooking time, different kinds of beans may vary in cooking time, then add the tomatoes and greens and serve immediately.) Before serving, stir in the chopped greens.

Serve over hot cooked rice, polenta, or with bread.

Makes a lot--enough for at least 10-12 servings. Freeze half for later or invite friends over.

Dirty Chai

Ingredients
1 1/4 cups non-dairy milk (I prefer soy)
1/2 cup freshly-brewed espresso or coffee
2 large orange peels
2 star anise
1 cinnamon stick
4 black or white peppercorns
6 drops vanilla stevia liquid and/or additional preferred sweetener to taste

Instructions
Put all ingredients in a small 1.5-quart slow cooker and set to low. Cook for 3-4 hours. You can also cook this on high for 2-3 hours.
Strain out the solids and discard. Serve.

Curried Vegetable & Chickpea Stew
Serves 8 to 10

Ingredients
1 teaspoon olive oil
1 large onion, diced
2 medium red or yellow potatoes, diced
1 tablespoon kosher salt
1 tablespoon curry powder
1 tablespoon brown sugar
1-inch piece ginger, peeled and grated
(about 1 tablespoon)
3 garlic cloves, minced
1/8 teaspoon cayenne pepper, optional
2 cups vegetable broth
2 (15.5-ounce) cans chickpeas, drained
and rinsed
1 green bell pepper, diced
1 red bell pepper, diced
1 medium head of cauliflower, cut into
bite-sized florets
1 (28-ounce) can diced tomatoes with
their juices
1/4 teaspoon black pepper
1 (10-ounce) bag baby spinach
1 cup coconut milk

Instructions

Heat the oil in a skillet over medium heat. Sauté the onion with one teaspoon of salt until translucent, about 5 minutes. Add the potatoes and another teaspoon of salt, and sauté until just translucent around the edges.

Stir in the curry, brown sugar, ginger, garlic, and chili and cook until fragrant, about 30 seconds. Pour in 1/4 cup of broth and scrape up any toasty bits from the bottom of the pan. Transfer this onion-potato mixture into the bowl of a 6-quart or larger slow cooker. (Halve this recipe for a smaller slow cooker.)

To the slow-cooker, add the rest of the broth, chickpeas, bell pepper, cauliflower, tomatoes with their juices, the pepper, and the final teaspoon of salt. Stir to combine. The liquid should come about half way up the sides of the bowl; add more broth as necessary. Cover and cook for 4 hours on HIGH.

Stir in the spinach and coconut milk. Cover with lid for a few more minutes to allow

the spinach to wilt. Taste and correct the salt and other seasonings as needed.
Serve on its own or over cous cous, Israeli cous cous, or orzo pasta.

Quick Oatmeal

Ingredients
2 cups old fashioned oats (I get this in bulk from my food co-op, if you used the quick cooking ones, it might be even creamier)
6 cups water, I think you need more than usual because of the long cooking time
cinnamon (optional)
dried fruits (optional)
spices (optional)

Directions
Put the oats and the water, along with anything else you want to add to the mix in the crock pot, turn on to low, and go to bed thinking about what a great breakfast you're going to have!

I scoop it out of the crock pot and eat it with maple syrup, or blueberry syrup, or pourable fruit, and soy milk--yum!

To reheat leftovers, I usually add a little water, and stir it a couple of times while microwaving until it's hot.

You can add other flavorings as you like, such as dried fruits, other sweet spices, diced apples, etc.

I usually put raisins on after it's cooked because I like them chewy.

I've been meaning to try dried cranberries.

Tofu in Pineapple BBQ Sauce

Ingredients
2 14-ounce packages extra-firm tofu, frozen and defrosted
1 large onion, chopped
8 large cloves garlic, minced
1/2 cup pitted dates (about 2.5 ounces)
1 1/2 cup crushed pineapple in own juice
1/3 cup water
2 fresh hot chile peppers, chopped

2 inches ginger-root, peeled and minced (about 3 tablespoons minced)
5 tablespoons tomato paste
2 tablespoons tamari or lite soy sauce
1 tablespoon lime juice
1 tablespoon cider vinegar
generous grating of black pepper
Salt, (optional), to taste

Instructions
At least 1 day before you plan to cook, place two packages of extra-firm tofu (water-pack style, not silken) into the freezer. Freeze at least 24 hours (this makes it firmer and sponge-like, which helps it hold up to long, slow cooking). Remove from freezer and allow to defrost in the refrigerator or use a quick defrost method (microwave or hot water bath). When tofu is completely defrosted, cut each block into halves horizontally and cut each half again vertically. Take each piece of tofu between your hands and gently press over a sink to squeeze out as much water as possible. Cut into 1/2-inch cubes.

Saute the onion in a non-stick pan (or on the browning setting, if your crock-pot has one) until it begins to brown. Add the garlic and cook for another minute. Scrape the onion/garlic into a blender and add all remaining ingredients except tofu and salt. Blend on high speed until sauce is a uniform consistency.

Place the tofu into the slow cooker (sprayed with non-stick spray or canola oil, if necessary) and pour the sauce over it. Stir very gently to make sure all sides of the tofu are covered. Cover and cook on Low for 8 hours or until sauce is absorbed and thickened. (Note: some crockpots run hotter than others so check once or twice to make sure the tofu isn't sticking or falling apart.) Check seasonings and add salt and extra lime juice as needed. Serve over salad greens.

Bean & Cornbread Casserole

Ingredients

1 green or red bell pepper

1 sweet or white onion

3 cloves garlic

1 can (15oz) red kidney beans, drained and rinsed

1 can (15oz) pinto beans, drained and rinsed

1 can (15oz) black beans, drained and rinsed

8-10oz tomato sauce

15 oz can diced tomatoes w/ chilies

1 can cream corn, halved

2 teaspoons chili powder

1 teaspoon pepper

2 teaspoon salt

1 teaspoon hot sauce

1/2 cup yellow corn meal

1/2 cup AP flour

1 1/4 teaspoon baking powder

1 teaspoon salt

1 tablespoon sugar

3/4 cup non-dairy milk

1 egg replacer mix of choice (I've used chia seeds, and I've also used banana-both worked!)

1 1/2 tablespoon vegetable oil

Instructions
Spray the inside of your slow cooker with non-stick spray.
Chop onions and bell peppers, and mince garlic cloves. Water saute over medium until tender, 6-8 minutes, then add to the slow-cooker. Add the beans, tomatoes, tomato sauce, 1/2 can of the creamed corn, spices and hot sauce. Mix, cover and cook on high for about 1 hour.
In a separate bowl, combine the cornmeal, flour, baking powder, salt and sugar, then stir in the milk, egg replacer, oil, and the rest of the creamed corn. Mix well.
Lade over the bean mixture in the slow cooker, making it nice and smooth.
Cover again, and cook for another 90 minutes on high (sometimes my cornbread takes another 30 minutes beyond that- just slice into yours to see if it's done!)

Muesli-Crock Pot

Ingredients
5 cups rolled oats
1 cup baking natural bran
1 cup wheat germ
1/2 cup coconut (desiccated, thread or slices)
1/2 cup raw sugar (white will not work)
4 tablespoons oil (I use olive)
2 teaspoons vanilla
Extras
sesame seeds
pumpkin seeds
sunflower seeds
peanuts
walnuts
linseeds, Use any mixture of the above up to 1 1/2
Dried fruit
raisins
sultana
currants
dried apricot
dried cherries
dried apple, etc. About 1/2 to 3/4 cup

Directions

Pre-heat the crock pot on high for 20 minutes.

Combine grains, seeds, nuts, sugar, oil and vanilla in the crock-pot.

Add the oil and vanilla and stir thoroughly.

Cover with lid and cook on high for about 2 hours stirring once or twice while cooking.

Remove lid after cooking is finished, stir thoroughly and allow to cool completely before stirring in the dried fruit and then storing in an air-tight container. The Tupperware cereal container is perfect.

Enjoy!

Lentil Chili

Serves: 12

Ingredients

1 tablespoon olive oil

2 medium onions, chopped

6-8 garlic cloves, minced

2 carrots, chopped

1 celery stalk, chopped

2 tablespoons chili powder

2 teaspoons cumin powder

1 teaspoon coriander powder

1 teaspoon dried oregano

1 teaspoon dry mustard

One 28-ounce box crushed tomatoes

salt to taste

One 16-ounce package dry lentils (I used brown lentils), picked through for stones, rinsed and drained

6-7 cups vegetable or chicken broth

Directions

Heat oil in a large pot. Add onions, garlic, carrots and celery. Saute until onions are softened and lightly browned, about 3-4 minutes. Add chili powder, cumin, coriander, oregano and mustard and stir well for a minute or two. Add tomatoes and salt to taste. Pour mixture into crockpot and add lentils and 6 cups of broth.

Cook for 4-6 hours. Add more broth or water as needed to achieve desired consistency.

Vegan Sin-Cinnati Chili

Ingredients
3/4 cup dry black beluga lentils (you can sub other lentils, the chili just won't be as dark)
1 1/2 cup water
1 1/2 cup diced tomatoes
2 cloves garlic, minced
1/2 cup Ground Beefless (use Trader Joe's, frozen crumbles, or cook 1/2 cup Gimme Lean)
1 bay leaf
1/2 teaspoon cumin
1/4 teaspoon ground hot pepper, like chipotle
1/8 teaspoon cinnamon
1 teaspoon chili powder
1 teaspoon cocoa

pinch allspice

pinch ground hot pepper of choice, optional and to taste

dash of freshly ground nutmeg

salt, to taste

shredded vegan cheese, for topping

chopped onions, for topping

cooked spinach pasta, for topping

Instructions

In the morning: Add everything except nutmeg, salt and toppings to the slow cooker . Cook 7 – 9 hours on low.

Pinto Beans & Rice

Ingredients

1 (1 lb) bag dried pinto bean

1/3 cup picante sauce

2 1/2 teaspoons salt

1/2 teaspoon pepper

1 teaspoon garlic powder

1 tablespoon garlic, minced (kind in jar is okay)
1 tablespoon chili powder
1/2 teaspoon cumin
1/2 teaspoon oregano
3 bay leaves
1 cup cooked white rice

Directions
Rinse beans in colander.
Put in a crock pot (or large pot).
Cover with water, plus about 2 inches over top of beans.
Add all ingredients, except rice.
Cook on high in crock pot about 3 hours til tender. (Crockpots vary greatly on cooking times. It could take much longer in yours, so the first time allow longer to cook and then you will know how long cooking time will be in the future.).
(Add water if necessary) May also cook on low overnight.
Add rice and cook until rice is warm.
Serve with cornbread.

Vegetarian Ratatouille

Ingredients
2 large onions, cut in half and sliced
1 large eggplant, sliced, cut in 2 inch pieces
4 small zucchini, sliced
2 garlic cloves, minced
2 large green bell peppers, de-seeded and cut into thin strips
2 large tomatoes, cut into 1/2 inch wedges
1 (6 ounce) cans tomato paste
1 teaspoon dried basil
1/2 teaspoon oregano
1 teaspoon sugar
2 teaspoons salt
1/2 teaspoon black pepper
2 tablespoons fresh parsley, chopped
1/4 cup olive oil
red pepper flakes, to spice it up

Directions
Layer half the vegetables in a large crock pot in the following order: onion, eggplant, zucchini, garlic, green peppers, tomatoes.

Next sprinkle half the basil, oregano, sugar, parsley, salt and pepper on the veggies.

Dot with half of the tomato paste.

Repeat layering process with remaining vegetables, spices and tomato paste.

Drizzle with olive oil.

Cover and cook on LOW for 7 to 9 hours.

Place in serving bowl and sprinkle with freshly grated Parmesan cheese.

Refrigerate to store.

Vegetarian Split Pea Soup

Ingredients
16 ounces split peas
4 medium carrots, peeled and diced
1 -1 1/2 cup white onion, chopped
2 garlic cloves, smashed
1 bay leaf
1 tablespoon salt
1/2 teaspoon pepper
6 cups hot water

Directions

Layer ingredients in order listed above. Do not stir

Cover and cook until peas are soft High: 4-5 hours or Low: 8-10 hours

Remove bay leaf and garlic (if it has held together) before serving.

Ratatouille With Chickpeas

Ingredients

1 tablespoon vegetable oil

1 onion, chopped

4 garlic cloves, minced

6 cups eggplants, cubed (one large)

2 teaspoons basil (dried)

1 teaspoon oregano (dried)

1/2 teaspoon salt

1/2 teaspoon pepper

1 red pepper

1 yellow pepper

2 zucchini

1/3 cup tomato paste
1 (19 ounce) cans chickpeas, drained and rinsed
1 (28 ounce) cans tomatoes
1/4 cup fresh basil or 1/4 cup fresh parsley, chopped

Directions
In a large skillet, heat oil over medium heat, cook onion, garlic, eggplant, basil, oregano, salt & pepper, stirring occasionally, until onion is softened, about 10 minutes. Scrape into crockpot.

Halve, core, and seed peppers; cut into 1 inch pieces. Cut zucchini into half lengthwise, cut crosswise into 1 1/2 inch chunks. Add to crockpot.

Add tomato paste, chickpeas, and tomatoes, breaking up tomatoes with a spoon. Cover and cook on low for 4 hours, or until vegetables are tender. Stir in basil / parsley.

Rice With Mangoes & Spicy Black Beans

Ingredients
1 tablespoon olive oil
1 small onion, finely chopped
1/2 red bell pepper, seeded and chopped
2 garlic cloves, minced
1 jalapeno, seeded and minced (any hot chile pepper okay)
1 teaspoon fresh ginger, peeled and minced
1/2 teaspoon ground cumin
1/2 teaspoon ground allspice
1/2 teaspoon dried oregano
2 (15 1/2 ounce) cans black beans, drained and rinsed
1 cup water
1/2 teaspoon light brown sugar
1/2 teaspoon salt
1/4 teaspoon black pepper, freshly ground
3 cups cooked long-grain brown rice (white rice okay)
2 mangoes, ripe, medium sized, peeled and flesh diced

Directions

Heat oil in large skillet over medium heat.

Add onion, bell pepper, garlic and jalapeno, cover, and cook 5 minutes until softened.

Add in seasonings, mix well and cook for 1 minute.

Transfer mixture into a 3 1/2 to 4 quart slow cooker.

Add bean, water, brown sugar, salt and pepper.

Stir well.

Cover and cook on low for 6 to 8 hours.

Add the cooked rice and the mangoes.

Allow to cook another 10 minutes.

Serve and enjoy.

Curry-Crock Pot

Ingredients

4 small potatoes, diced or 4 small potatoes, chunked

2 (14 ounce) cans Rotel tomatoes & chilies

2 (15 1/2 ounce) cans kidney beans or 2
(15 1/2 ounce) cans chickpeas
2 white onions, chopped
2 tablespoons olive oil
1 tablespoon good quality curry powder
1 teaspoon cayenne (optional)
1/2 teaspoon cardamom (optional)
1/2 teaspoon ginger (optional)

Directions

Heat olive oil in a saucepan or skillet. Add spices, saute for 1 minute or so.

Add onions and saute for 2 - 5 minutes.

Add both cans of Rotel.

Pour mixture into crockpot. Add potatoes and canned beans to crockpot.

Allow to crock on low for 6 - 9 hours or on high for 3 - 5 hours, depending on your crockpot.

Serve over rice or with makki di roti (indian cornbread).

Tomato Spinach Soup

Ingredients
10 ounces Baby Spinach, washed
2 medium carrots, chopped
2 medium celery ribs, chopped
1 large onion, chopped
1 garlic clove, minced
4 cups low sodium vegetable broth
1 (28 ounce) diced tomatoes
2 leaves bay leaves
1 tablespoon dried basil
1 teaspoon dried oregano
1/2 teaspoon red pepper flakes, crushed

Directions
Place all ingredients in a slow cooker.
Cover and cook on high for 5 hours or low
for 8-10 hours.
Remove bay leaves, stir and serve.
Yields about 1 cup per serving.

Vegetarian Chipotle Chili

Ingredients

1 (15 ounce) cans black beans, drained and rinsed (or 1 1/2 - 2 cups cooked beans)
1 (15 ounce) cans navy beans, drained and rinsed (or 1 1/2 - 2 cups cooked beans)
1 (14 1/2 ounce) cans diced tomatoes
1 (14 1/2 ounce) cans diced tomatoes and green chilies or 1 (14 1/2 ounce) cans diced tomatoes with jalapenos
1 cup onion, chopped
6 garlic cloves, minced
2 tablespoons chili powder
1 tablespoon sweet Hungarian paprika
1 tablespoon dried cilantro (optional)
1/2 teaspoon fresh coarse ground black pepper
1 teaspoon chipotle chile, minced

Directions

Stir everything together in a 4 1/2 quart or larger slow cooker.
Set power to low and cook for 6 hours or longer (we usually let this cook for 10 hours).

Serve with cheese or sour cream if you wish.

Vegetarian Spaghetti Sauce

Ingredients
2 tablespoons olive oil
1 onion, chopped
2 carrots, peeled and chopped
2 cups sliced mushrooms
1 green bell pepper, chopped
2 (14 ounce) cans diced tomatoes with seasonings, undrained
15 ounces tomato sauce
6 ounces tomato paste
2 teaspoons sugar
1/2 teaspoon salt
1/4 teaspoon pepper
12 ounces spaghetti
parmesan cheese (optional)

Directions

Cook onions and carrots in oil in large nonstick skillet over medium heat.

Stir and cook for 4-5 minutes until tender. Add mushrooms and bell pepper and stir.

Place vegetables into bottom of 4-5 quart crock pot and add remaining ingredients except spaghetti pasta and cheese.

Cover crock pot and cook on low for 7-8 hours.

Uncover, stir thoroughly, then leave cover off crock pot and turn heat to high.

Cook, uncovered, for 1 more hour to thicken sauce.

At this point the sauce can be frozen. Divide into smaller portions and cool in refrigerator.

Wrap, label, and freeze the sauce up to 3 months.

To thaw and reheat, thaw sauce overnight in refrigerator.

Pour into skillet and heat over medium heat, stirring frequently, about 15-20 minutes or until sauce bubbles and is thoroughly heated.

You can even cook the pasta until almost tender and combine it with the cooled sauce. Freeze as directed, and thaw as directed. You may need to add 1/4-1/3 cup water when reheating if freezing the pasta in the sauce.

Or you can go ahead and serve sauce with cooked spaghetti and grated Parmesan cheese. 6 servings.

Split Pea Soup

Ingredients
6 cups water
2 cups split peas, rinsed and picked over
1 stalk celery, coarsely chopped
1 large carrot, chopped
1 medium onion, chopped
1/4 teaspoon thyme
1 dash red pepper
1 bay leaf
salt
pepper

Directions

Combine water, peas, celery, carrot, onion, thyme, red pepper and bay leaf in crock pot.

Season to taste with salt and pepper.

Cook on low until split peas and vegetables are tender (anywhere from 6-8 hours).

Press soup through fine sieve and reheat just to boiling point or use hand blender to smooth.

Spicy Lentil Soup

Ingredients
1/4 cup extra virgin olive oil
1 large onion (dice half and chop the other half)
kosher salt, to taste
black pepper, to taste
1 -2 teaspoon crushed red pepper flakes
3 large celery ribs, chopped
3 carrots, chopped
2 garlic cloves (minced)

1 cup chopped cauliflower
2 teaspoons curry powder
1 teaspoon cumin
16 ounces dry lentils
1 (14 1/2 ounce) cans vegetable broth
2 (14 1/2 ounce) cans diced tomatoes with juice
8 cups water
2 teaspoons cayenne pepper

Directions

Heat 1/4 cup olive oil in a large pot over medium-low heat. Add onions, salt, pepper, and crushed red pepper, cover and simmer for 6 minutes, or until onions are clear and soft.

(If using the crockpot, you would now transfer the onion mixture to your crockpot, add all other dry and liquid ingredients and give it a good stir, and cook on LOW for 8 hours until the lentils are soft. If using the stovetop, please continue to step 3.).

Add celery, carrots, garlic, cauliflower, curry, and cumin, and stir. Cover and let simmer for 10 minutes, stirring occasionally.

Stir in lentils, vegetable broth and tomatoes. Cover and let simmer for another 10 minutes, stirring occasionally.

Add 8 cups of water and increase to high heat, and leave uncovered until it begins to boil.

When the soup comes to a boil, reduce heat and add cayenne pepper. Let simmer for at least 2 hours, or until lentils are soft.

Thyme Roasted Beets

Ingredients
12 beets (about 2 bunches)
4 garlic cloves, minced
2 tablespoons olive oil
1 teaspoon dried thyme
1/2 teaspoon salt
1/2 teaspoon pepper
1 tablespoon minced fresh rosemary or 1 tablespoon fresh parsley

Directions

Peel and dice the beets, then place in crock pot.

Add garlic, 1/4 cup water, oil, thyme, salt and pepper.

Stir all ingredients until well combined.

Cover and cook for 6 hours on low until tender.

Sprinkle with parsley.

Sweet Potato Chili

Ingredients

1 medium onion, diced

1 medium zucchini, halved lengthways and then sliced into pieces about 1/4-inch thick

1 large sweet potato (chopped into bite sized pieces...use yam if you prefer)

1 (15 ounce) cans white beans (aka Great Northern beans)

1 (14 ounce) cans tomato sauce (a slightly smaller can or jar....ie 10oz is OK too)

1 (15 ounce) cans diced tomatoes

2 tablespoons chili powder (can add about 1/2 tsp more if you like it really hot)

2 tablespoons brown sugar

1 1/2 teaspoons curry powder

2 teaspoons ground cumin

1/4 teaspoon pepper

1/2 teaspoon cinnamon

1/2 lb butternut squash, peeled and cut into 1-inch chunks

1/2 lb fresh green beans, trimmed and cut into 2-inch pieces

1 teaspoon red wine vinegar

1/2 teaspoon sea salt

Directions

Place all ingredients into crockpot, stir gently.

Cook about 5 hours on high or 8-10 on low.

Vegetarian Unbeef Stew

Ingredients

1 lb extra firm tofu

1 large onion, chopped

1 quart vegetable broth

3 -5 tablespoons vegan worcestershire sauce

1 tablespoon tamari (soy sauce)

2 garlic cloves, finely chopped

4 large carrots, peeled and chopped

4 large potatoes, peeled and chopped

1/2 cup sliced celery

1 tomatoes, seeded and diced

1 1/2 teaspoons salt

1/2 teaspoon black pepper

1 teaspoon basil

3 tablespoons soy margarine

3 -5 tablespoons cornstarch, mixed with water until no longer lumpy

Directions

Wrap and freeze the tofu and then let it thaw out completely. Drain the water from the tofu, and cut into slices. Press out any remaining water. Cut the slices into chunks and bake at 200°F on an ungreased cookie sheet while chopping the rest of the ingredients; check the tofu about every 10 to 15 minutes so that it doesn't get browned--it should just be dried out, not burned. The tofu should be well dried out, like croutons.

Place all of the prepared ingredients into a crockpot, stir well, and cook on high for at least 6 to 8 hours, stirring occasionally. The stew is ready when it is thick and brown, and the vegetables are fork tender.

To press water from tofu:.

Place tofu block between two dinner plates. Place a heavy object, such as a cast iron pan, on top of the plates and wait for 15 minutes or so. Drain water from plates. Flip tofu block over and replace the plates. Place the cast iron pot on top on the plates once again. Drain for 15 minutes more. Discard water. Tofu is now ready to use, or can be placed in a plastic bag. Once bagged, place in the fridge until needed.

I usually press and drain the tofu when purchased, storing it in a plastic bag in the fridge so it will be ready to use when needed.

(Preparation time given above does not include pressing tofu).

Vegetarian Lentil Soup

Ingredients
1 lb green lentil
1 quart vegetable broth
4 cups water
4 celery ribs, diced
4 carrots, peeled and diced
1 onion, diced
6 -8 garlic cloves, minced
1 (14 ounce) cans diced tomatoes
1 teaspoon dried oregano
3 sprigs fresh thyme
2 bay leaves
1 pinch cayenne pepper
salt and pepper
1/2 lb Baby Spinach, roughly chopped

Directions
Combine all ingredients except spinach in crock pot. Cook on low heat for 8-10

hours, or until lentils have cooked and soup has thickened.

Stir in spinach and let sit, covered, a few minutes until spinach has completely wilted.

About the Author

Martin Bown is author of several cookbooks on Vegan diet. He has written research papers on the topic and currently lives in California.